HEALING TOUCH THERAPY FOR HEALTH

Comprehensive Guide To Pain Relief, Stress Reduction, And Enhanced Well-Being Through Energy Recovering Techniques

DR. MELISSA STOTLER

Copyright © 2023 by Dr. Melissa Stotler

Disclaimer:

The data in this book, "Acupuncture Therapy Simplified," is solely meant to be informative and instructional.

This book is not intended to replace expert medical advice, diagnosis, or care. No medical, health, or other professional services are offered by the author, publisher, or any affiliated parties

Individual outcomes may differ in the practice of these therapies, which entail a variety of approaches and methodologies.

A one-on-one session with a trained or certified healthcare professional is still preferable. It is best to consult a trained healthcare provider before making any decisions regarding your health.

The author of this book is not affiliated with any specific website, product, or organization related to any of these therapies.

All reasonable measures have been taken by the author and publisher to guarantee the authenticity and dependability of the material contained in this book.

Contents

CHAPTER ONE 21

THE SCIENCE BEHIND HEALING TOUCH
...................................21

Energy Fields And The Human Body.21

How Healing Touch Affects The Body22

Research Studies And Findings.......24

The Body's Natural Healing Processes
...................................25

Case Studies And Testimonials.......27

CHAPTER TWO..........................31

BASIC TECHNIQUES AND PRACTICES IN HEALING TOUCH THERAPY 31

Grounding And Centering 31

Clearing And Balancing Energy.......32

Chakra Alignment.....................33

Hands-On and Hands-Off Methods ...34

Self-Care Techniques For Practitioners
...................................35

CHAPTER THREE 37

HEALING TOUCH SESSIONS 37

Preparing For A Session 37

Gathering Necessary Tools 38

Conducting A Session Step-By-Step.39

Post-Session Practices 42

Client-Practitioner Communication...44

Maintaining Professional Boundaries.46

CHAPTER FOUR................................49

ADVANCED HEALING TOUCH METHODS
....49

Deepening Your Practice................49

Working With Complex Cases.........50

Integrating Other Modalities 51

Distance Healing Touch 53

Advanced Energy Field Interventions54

CHAPTER FIVE 57

HEALING TOUCH FOR SPECIFIC CONDITIONS 57

Pain Management 57

Stress And Anxiety Relief 58

Enhancing Recovery From Illness 60

Supporting Mental Health 61

Special Populations (Children, Elderly, Etc.) 62

CHAPTER SIX 65

DEVELOPING YOUR SKILLS 65

Continuing Education Opportunities .65

Workshops And Seminars 66

Mentorship And Community Support 67

Building A Practice.........................68

Reflective Practices For Growth 69

CHAPTER SEVEN 71

COMMON CONCERNS IN HEALING TOUCH THERAPY 71

Addressing Skepticism 71

Managing Client Expectations..........72

Handling Adverse Reactions.............73

Ethical Dilemmas And Solutions 74

Legal Considerations And Insurance.75

CHAPTER EIGHT 77

FREQUENTLY ASKED QUESTIONS (FAQS) 77

What Is Healing Touch Therapy? 77

How Does It Differ From Other Therapies? 78

What Can I Expect During A Session? 80

Is Healing Touch Suitable For Everyone? 81

How Do I Find A Qualified Practitioner? 82

Healing Touch Therapy for Health: A Beginner's Guide serves as an essential resource for anyone looking to understand and practice this transformative healing modality. The book begins with a thorough exploration of the history and background of Healing Touch Therapy, tracing its origins and development, highlighting influential figures, and detailing the evolution of techniques. This foundational knowledge is crucial for appreciating how Healing Touch has integrated into modern healthcare, supported by recognized organizations and certifications that lend credibility to the practice.

Delving into the science behind Healing Touch, this guide explains the intricate relationship between energy fields and the human body, shedding light on how Healing Touch affects the body's natural healing processes. It presents compelling research studies and findings that validate the practice, complemented by case studies and testimonials that illustrate real-world applications and outcomes. Understanding these scientific principles equips readers with a solid grounding in the efficacy and mechanisms of Healing Touch.

The book offers a practical guide to basic techniques and practices essential for beginners. Readers will learn the fundamentals of grounding and centering, clearing and balancing energy, and chakra alignment. It details both hands-on and hands-off methods, empowering practitioners with a versatile skill set. Self-care techniques are also emphasized, ensuring that practitioners maintain their well-being while helping others.

In the Healing Touch sessions section, the guide provides a comprehensive overview of how to prepare for, conduct, and follow up after a session. It emphasizes the importance of client-practitioner communication and maintaining professional boundaries, ensuring ethical and effective practice. This section is designed to build confidence in new practitioners, offering step-by-step instructions and best practices.

For those looking to advance their practice, the book explores advanced Healing Touch methods, including working with complex cases, integrating other modalities, and performing distance Healing Touch.

Advanced energy field interventions are also covered, providing depth and sophistication to the practitioner's toolkit.

The guide addresses the application of Healing Touch for specific conditions, such as pain management, stress and anxiety relief, and enhancing recovery from illness.

It also covers support for mental health and special populations like children and the elderly, showcasing the versatility and adaptability of Healing Touch.

Developing your skills is another key focus, with insights into continuing education opportunities, workshops, seminars, and mentorship.

Building a practice and engaging in reflective practices for growth are also discussed, helping practitioners to continually evolve and enhance their capabilities.

Addressing common concerns is critical for new practitioners. The book provides strategies for managing skepticism, handling client expectations, and dealing with adverse reactions. It also covers ethical dilemmas, solutions, and legal considerations, ensuring practitioners are well-prepared for all aspects of their practice.

Finally, a section dedicated to frequently asked questions (FAQs) offers clear answers to common queries about Healing Touch Therapy, its differentiation from other therapies, what to expect during a session, suitability for various individuals, and how to find a qualified practitioner.

This comprehensive FAQ section serves as a quick reference guide for both new and experienced practitioners.

History and Background of Healing Touch Therapy

Origins and Development

Healing Touch Therapy (HTT) is a relatively modern practice, tracing its roots back to the 1980s. The therapy emerged from the nursing field, specifically through the work of Janet Mentgen, a nurse with a profound interest in energy-based healing.

Mentgen combined her knowledge of nursing with various traditional healing practices to develop a systematic approach to energy healing. This approach aimed to balance and harmonize the human energy field, promoting physical, mental, and emotional well-being.

HTT draws upon ancient healing traditions from diverse cultures, including Chinese medicine, Ayurvedic practices, and indigenous healing methods. These traditions emphasize the importance of energy flow within the body, positing that health issues arise when this flow is disrupted. By incorporating these principles, Mentgen and her colleagues created a structured method that could be taught and applied within a clinical setting, making energy healing accessible and standardized for modern healthcare professionals.

Influential Figures in the Field

Several key figures have been instrumental in the development and popularization of Healing Touch Therapy. Janet Mentgen is widely regarded as the founder and primary visionary behind HTT. Her dedication to integrating energy healing into nursing practice laid the foundation for what has become a widely respected therapeutic modality.

Following Mentgen, other notable figures such as Alice McGurrin and Dorothea Hover-Kramer contributed significantly to the field. McGurrin expanded the scope of HTT by incorporating it into her work with patients, thereby demonstrating its practical benefits in clinical settings. Hover-Kramer, on the other hand, was pivotal in promoting HTT through her writings and educational efforts, helping to establish a broader acceptance and understanding of the therapy.

Evolution of Techniques

Over the years, the techniques used in Healing Touch Therapy have evolved and diversified. Initially, HTT focused on basic hand positions and simple energy interventions. Practitioners would use their hands to assess and influence the energy field surrounding the body, aiming to clear blockages and restore balance.

As the field grew, more sophisticated methods were developed. Techniques such as Magnetic Passes, Chakra Connection, and Chelation became standard practices within HTT. These methods involve a deeper understanding of the body's energy centers and pathways, allowing practitioners to address specific issues more effectively. Continuous research and feedback from practitioners have further refined these techniques, ensuring that HTT remains a dynamic and evolving field.

Integration into Modern Healthcare

Healing Touch Therapy has gradually found its place within modern healthcare systems. Initially met with skepticism, HTT has gained recognition and acceptance due to its demonstrated benefits and the advocacy of dedicated professionals. Today, many hospitals and clinics incorporate HTT as part of their integrative medicine programs, recognizing its potential to enhance patient care and support healing.

HTT is often used alongside conventional medical treatments, providing a complementary approach that addresses the whole person. Patients undergoing surgery, cancer treatments, or dealing with chronic pain have reported significant improvements in their overall well-being when HTT is included in their care plan. This integration underscores the therapy's versatility and effectiveness, as well as its alignment with the holistic health movement that emphasizes the interconnectedness of body, mind, and spirit.

Recognized Organizations and Certifications

The credibility and standardization of Healing Touch Therapy are supported by several recognized organizations and certification programs. The Healing Touch Program (HTP), founded by Janet Mentgen, remains one of the most prominent and respected organizations in the field. HTP offers a comprehensive certification process that ensures practitioners meet high standards of competence and professionalism.

Other organizations, such as Healing Beyond Borders (HBB), also play a vital role in promoting HTT. HBB provides education, resources, and certification for practitioners, fostering a global community committed to the practice and advancement of energy healing.

These organizations are instrumental in maintaining the integrity of HTT, offering ongoing education and support to ensure practitioners can deliver the highest quality care.

By providing standardized training and certification, these organizations help to ensure that HTT practitioners are well-prepared to integrate their skills into various healthcare settings.

This professionalization of HTT not only enhances its legitimacy but also ensures that patients receive safe and effective care from qualified practitioners.

CHAPTER ONE

THE SCIENCE BEHIND HEALING TOUCH

Energy Fields And The Human Body

The concept of energy fields around the human body is foundational to Healing Touch therapy. In various ancient traditions, this energy is known as "chi" in Chinese medicine, "prana" in Ayurveda, and "biofield" in Western complementary medicine. These energy fields are believed to flow around and through the body, creating a complex, dynamic network that influences physical, emotional, and spiritual health. Modern science is beginning to explore these fields with instruments like magnetometers and electrophotonic imaging, which suggest that our bodies emit and interact with subtle energies.

These energy fields can become disrupted by stress, trauma, or illness, leading to imbalances that manifest as physical symptoms or emotional disturbances. Healing Touch practitioners work to restore balance by using their hands to manipulate the energy fields. They believe that by clearing blockages and enhancing energy flow, the body's inherent ability to heal itself is activated.

How Healing Touch Affects The Body

Healing Touch aims to promote healing on multiple levels. Practitioners use their hands in a gentle, non-invasive manner, either lightly touching or hovering over the body. This interaction is thought to realign and balance the energy fields, which can lead to a cascade of physiological responses.

One immediate effect often reported by patients is a deep sense of relaxation. This relaxation response can reduce stress, which is known to have numerous negative effects on the body, including weakened immune function, elevated blood pressure, and disrupted sleep patterns.

By inducing relaxation, Healing Touch can help lower stress hormones, enhance immune function, and improve overall well-being.

Furthermore, Healing Touch is believed to enhance the body's natural healing processes. It may stimulate the production of endorphins and other neurotransmitters that promote a sense of well-being and pain relief. Some studies also suggest that it can improve circulation and oxygenation of tissues, facilitating the body's repair mechanisms.

Research Studies And Findings

Scientific interest in Healing Touch has grown in recent years, with various studies exploring its effectiveness. Research has shown that Healing Touch can be beneficial for a wide range of conditions, from anxiety and depression to chronic pain and cancer-related fatigue.

For example, a study published in the Journal of Alternative and Complementary Medicine found that Healing Touch significantly reduced anxiety and increased relaxation in patients undergoing radiation therapy. Another study in the International Journal of Nursing Studies reported that Healing Touch improved the quality of life and reduced pain in cancer patients.

Research also indicates that Healing Touch can positively impact physiological parameters. A randomized controlled trial demonstrated that patients who received Healing Touch had lower blood pressure and heart rate variability, indicating a stress reduction.

Moreover, another study found that Healing Touch enhanced immune function by increasing levels of salivary immunoglobulin A, an antibody that plays a critical role in mucosal immunity.

The Body's Natural Healing Processes

The human body possesses an extraordinary ability to heal itself, a process that can be enhanced by Healing Touch.

Our bodies are constantly in a state of repair and renewal, from the cellular level to entire organ systems. Healing Touch works by supporting these natural processes, providing the conditions necessary for optimal healing.

At the cellular level, Healing Touch can stimulate the repair and regeneration of tissues.

By promoting relaxation and reducing stress, it helps to lower levels of cortisol, a stress hormone that can inhibit healing. Additionally, it enhances blood flow and oxygen delivery to tissues, which are essential for cellular repair and growth.

On a systemic level, Healing Touch supports the body's immune response. The immune system is our primary defense against illness and injury, and its effectiveness can be compromised by stress and energy imbalances. By balancing the energy fields, Healing Touch can help boost immune function, making the body more resilient to infections and diseases.

Case Studies And Testimonials

Numerous case studies and testimonials highlight the benefits of Healing Touch. These personal stories provide compelling evidence of its effectiveness and the profound impact it can have on individuals' lives.

One case involves a woman suffering from chronic migraines. Traditional treatments had little effect, but after several Healing Touch sessions, she reported a significant reduction in the frequency and severity of her migraines. She described the sessions as deeply relaxing and felt that they addressed not just her physical pain but also underlying emotional stress.

Another testimonial comes from a cancer patient undergoing chemotherapy. He experienced severe nausea and fatigue, which conventional treatments could not fully alleviate.

After incorporating Healing Touch into his care regimen, he noticed a remarkable improvement in his symptoms.

He felt more energetic and less nauseous, which greatly enhanced his quality of life during a challenging time.

A child with severe anxiety also benefited from Healing Touch. Traditional therapies had limited success, but after several sessions of Healing Touch, her anxiety levels decreased dramatically.

She became more calm and focused, and her parents observed a significant improvement in her overall behavior and emotional well-being.

These case studies and testimonials illustrate the potential of Healing Touch to transform lives. By tapping into the body's natural healing abilities and addressing the energetic imbalances that contribute to illness, Healing Touch offers a holistic approach to health and well-being.

CHAPTER TWO

BASIC TECHNIQUES AND PRACTICES IN HEALING TOUCH THERAPY

Grounding And Centering

Grounding and centering are foundational practices in healing touch therapy, essential for both practitioners and recipients. Grounding connects you to the Earth, creating a sense of stability and balance. To ground yourself, start by standing or sitting comfortably, ensuring your feet are flat on the ground. Visualize roots extending from the soles of your feet deep into the Earth. Feel the energy of the Earth rising through these roots, bringing stability and strength.

Centering, on the other hand, focuses on aligning your energy to a central point within your body, usually around the solar plexus or heart area. This process helps you stay calm and focused, especially during a healing session. To center yourself, close your eyes and take deep, calming breaths. Visualize a point of light in your chosen area (solar plexus or heart) and feel it expand with each breath, radiating calm and balanced energy throughout your body.

Clearing And Balancing Energy

Clearing and balancing energy involves removing blockages and restoring the natural flow of energy within the body. Blocked or stagnant energy can cause physical and emotional discomfort, so this practice is crucial in healing touch therapy. To clear energy, you can use techniques such as sweeping motions with your hands above the body or using visualizations.

For instance, imagine a gentle stream of water washing away any negative or stagnant energy from the body. As you perform sweeping motions with your hands, visualize this stream carrying away the blockages, leaving the energy pathways clear. Balancing energy involves ensuring that energy is evenly distributed throughout the body. You can use your hands to sense areas with excess or deficient energy and then move energy accordingly to create balance.

Chakra Alignment

Chakra alignment focuses on the body's seven main energy centers, known as chakras, which run along the spine from the base to the crown of the head. Each chakra corresponds to different physical, emotional, and spiritual aspects of our being. To align the chakras, begin by visualizing each chakra as a spinning wheel of light in its respective color: red for the root chakra, orange for the sacral chakra, yellow for the solar plexus chakra, green for the heart chakra, blue for the throat chakra, indigo for the third eye chakra, and violet for the crown chakra.

Using your hands, move in a clockwise motion over each chakra, visualizing them spinning harmoniously and brightly. This helps clear any blockages and ensures each chakra is aligned and functioning optimally. Regular chakra alignment can promote overall well-being and balance in the body.

Hands-On and Hands-Off Methods

Healing touch therapy employs both hands-on and hands-off methods, depending on the practitioner's preference and the recipient's comfort level. Hands-on methods involve light touch on specific areas of the body to transfer healing energy directly. For instance, placing hands on the shoulders, back, or feet can help channel energy to those areas.

Hands-off methods, on the other hand, involve working with the energy field surrounding the body. This can include techniques such as sweeping motions above the body, sending energy through intention and visualization, or using pendulums to detect and clear energy imbalances. Both methods are effective, and the choice often depends on the practitioner's training and the specific needs of the recipient.

Self-Care Techniques For Practitioners

Self-care is vital for healing touch practitioners to maintain their energy levels and prevent burnout. Regular grounding and centering are essential practices, as mentioned earlier.

Additionally, practitioners should engage in activities that replenish their energy, such as spending time in nature, meditating, and practicing yoga or tai chi.

Proper hydration, a balanced diet, and sufficient rest are also crucial for maintaining physical and energetic health.

Practitioners can also benefit from receiving healing touch sessions themselves to clear any accumulated energy imbalances. By prioritizing self-care, practitioners ensure they can provide effective and compassionate care to their clients.

CHAPTER THREE

HEALING TOUCH SESSIONS

Preparing For A Session

Creating a Healing Environment

Before a Healing Touch session begins, it is crucial to establish a serene and inviting environment. This involves selecting a quiet space free from distractions where both the practitioner and client can focus entirely on the session.

The room should be clean, well-ventilated, and comfortably warm. Soft lighting can help create a calming atmosphere; consider using dimmable lights or candles.

Aromatherapy, with scents like lavender or chamomile, can further enhance relaxation, but ensure the client does not have any allergies or sensitivities.

Gathering Necessary Tools

Preparation also involves assembling all the necessary tools and materials. A comfortable massage table or chair should be prepared with clean linens.

Practitioners might also use bolsters or pillows to ensure the client's comfort. Additionally, having water and tissues nearby can be helpful. Tools like tuning forks, crystals, or specific oils might be used depending on the practitioner's methods and the client's needs. Always ensure that hands are clean and that any tools are sanitized before the session begins.

Setting Intentions

Setting a clear intention is a pivotal part of preparing for a Healing Touch session. Both the practitioner and the client should take a moment to focus on what they hope to achieve during the session. This could be specific physical healing, emotional release, or overall energy balancing. Taking a few deep breaths together and perhaps sharing these intentions can help align both parties and create a cooperative energy flow. Grounding exercises, such as visualizing roots extending from the feet into the earth, can help both practitioner and client feel centered and present.

Conducting A Session Step-By-Step

Initial Consultation

Each session begins with a brief consultation to discuss the client's current state and specific concerns. This dialogue helps the practitioner tailor the session to the client's needs. Questions about physical health, emotional well-being, and any particular issues should be asked. This also establishes trust and opens a line of communication that will be essential throughout the session.

Energy Assessment

The practitioner will typically begin with an energy assessment to understand the client's energetic field. This can be done through techniques such as hand scanning, where the practitioner moves their hands a few inches above the client's body to sense any imbalances. This initial scan helps identify areas that need attention and can guide the focus of the session.

Healing Techniques

The actual healing techniques used in a session can vary widely but generally involve the practitioner using their hands to clear, balance, and energize the client's energy field. This might include light touch or hands hovering just above the body. Techniques such as chakra balancing, energy channeling, and specific hand movements are commonly used. The practitioner might move their hands in sweeping motions to clear negative energy or place them on specific areas to transfer positive energy. Throughout the session, the practitioner remains attentive to the flow of energy and any shifts that occur.

Closing the Session

Closing the session is as important as the opening. The practitioner will often perform a final energy sweep to ensure the client's energy field is balanced and clear. Afterward, the client is given a few moments to rest and integrate the healing before slowly sitting up. Offering water and gently discussing the client's experience can help ground them back into their physical body and the present moment.

Post-Session Practices

Immediate Aftercare

Once the session is concluded, it's essential to address immediate aftercare. Clients should be encouraged to take their time getting up, as the energy shifts can sometimes cause lightheadedness or disorientation. Providing a glass of water and recommending a few minutes of quiet reflection can aid in grounding the energy.

Self-Care Recommendations

Providing clients with self-care recommendations helps extend the benefits of the session. This might include suggestions for gentle activities like walking, yoga, or meditation.

Encouraging clients to stay hydrated and perhaps take a salt bath can help in detoxifying and grounding their energy. Recommending specific affirmations or mindfulness exercises tailored to the client's needs can also be beneficial.

Follow-Up

Follow-up is an integral part of post-session care. Practitioners should check in with clients within a few days to discuss any experiences or changes they've noticed.

This follow-up can be done through a phone call, email, or another preferred method. It helps the practitioner understand the session's impact and make any necessary adjustments for future sessions.

Client-Practitioner Communication

Establishing Open Communication

Effective communication between the client and practitioner is crucial for a successful Healing Touch session.

From the first consultation, it's important to establish a rapport and ensure that the client feels comfortable expressing their concerns and expectations.

Practitioners should listen actively, show empathy, and validate the client's experiences. This creates a trusting environment where the client feels safe and understood.

Explaining the Process

Clients often benefit from understanding what to expect during a session. Practitioners should take time to explain the techniques and processes involved, addressing any questions or concerns the client may have.

This helps alleviate any anxiety and sets clear expectations. Informing the client about sensations they might feel during the session, such as warmth, tingling, or emotional release, prepares them for the experience.

Feedback During the Session

During the session, maintaining an open line of communication is essential. Practitioners should periodically check in with the client to ensure their comfort and to gauge their reactions to the treatment.

This can be done subtly, by asking simple questions about how they feel or if they are comfortable. Adjustments can be made based on the client's feedback to enhance their experience.

Maintaining Professional Boundaries

Defining Boundaries

Maintaining professional boundaries is fundamental in Healing Touch therapy. Clear boundaries help protect both the client and practitioner, ensuring a respectful and professional relationship.

Practitioners should establish these boundaries from the first interaction, outlining the scope of the session and what the client can expect. This includes discussing the nature of physical touch and obtaining explicit consent.

Respecting Personal Space

Respecting the client's personal space is crucial. Practitioners should always ask for permission before placing their hands on the client's body and explaining the purpose of each touch.

If a client is uncomfortable with any aspect of the session, it is the practitioner's responsibility to adapt and respect their wishes. Ensuring the client feels in control of their own experience fosters trust and safety.

Handling Emotional Releases

Healing Touch sessions can often lead to emotional releases. Practitioners need to handle these with sensitivity and professionalism.

Providing a safe space for clients to express their emotions without judgment is essential.

Practitioners should offer support, such as tissues or a comforting presence, but also know when to give the client space.

Offering to refer clients to additional support services, such as counseling, can be beneficial if deeper emotional issues arise.

Ongoing Education and Supervision

Practitioners should engage in ongoing education and seek supervision to maintain professional boundaries and enhance their practice. Regularly attending workshops, training, and peer supervision helps practitioners stay informed about best practices and ethical guidelines.

This commitment to professional development ensures that they provide the highest standard of care while maintaining appropriate boundaries.

CHAPTER FOUR

ADVANCED HEALING TOUCH METHODS

Deepening Your Practice

To deepen your practice in Healing Touch Therapy, it's essential to move beyond the basics and immerse yourself in advanced techniques and principles. Begin by refining your skills through consistent practice, focusing on your sensitivity to energy fields and your ability to channel healing energy effectively. Participate in advanced training workshops and seek mentorship from experienced practitioners to gain new insights and feedback on your techniques.

Developing a deeper connection with your clients is also crucial. Spend time understanding their unique needs and energy patterns. This can involve detailed consultations and energy assessments to tailor your approach to each individual. By cultivating a deeper sense of empathy and intuition, you'll be able to identify subtle energy imbalances and address them more effectively.

Working With Complex Cases

Working with complex cases in Healing Touch Therapy requires a comprehensive understanding of both the physical and energetic aspects of health.

These cases often involve chronic conditions, severe trauma, or multiple health issues. Start by conducting a thorough assessment of the client's energy field, noting areas of blockage, depletion, or excess energy.

Incorporate a holistic approach by considering the client's emotional, mental, and spiritual well-being alongside their physical health. Use advanced techniques such as energy clearing, balancing, and re-patterning to address deep-seated issues. Collaboration with other healthcare professionals can also be beneficial, ensuring a comprehensive care plan that supports the client's overall healing journey.

Documenting your sessions meticulously is essential when dealing with complex cases. Keep detailed records of the client's progress, noting any changes in their energy field and overall health. This will help you adjust your techniques as needed and provide valuable insights for future sessions.

Integrating Other Modalities

Integrating other healing modalities with Healing Touch Therapy can enhance the effectiveness of your practice and offer a more comprehensive approach to health and wellness. Consider incorporating practices such as Reiki, acupuncture, aromatherapy, or chiropractic care, which can complement Healing Touch techniques.

Begin by familiarizing yourself with the basics of these modalities and understanding how they interact with energy healing. For example, combining Healing Touch with acupuncture can help to balance the body's energy meridians, while aromatherapy can enhance the healing environment and promote relaxation.

Develop a personalized approach for each client, selecting the most appropriate modalities based on their specific needs. Always communicate clearly with your clients about the techniques you are using and ensure they are comfortable with the integrated approach. Continuous education and collaboration with practitioners from other fields can also expand your knowledge and improve your practice.

Distance Healing Touch

Distance Healing Touch, also known as remote healing, involves sending healing energy to someone who is not physically present. This advanced technique requires a strong connection to the universal energy field and a high level of focus and intention.

To perform Distance Healing Touch, begin by centering yourself and setting a clear intention for the healing session. Visualize the person you are working with and their energy field. Use your hands to direct energy to specific areas of your body, just as you would in an in-person session. Techniques such as visualization, intention setting, and guided imagery can enhance the effectiveness of distance healing.

Establishing a clear communication channel with your client is crucial. Before the session, discuss their needs and concerns, and guide how they can prepare. After the session, follow up to discuss any sensations or changes they experienced. Consistent practice and feedback from clients will help you refine your distance healing skills.

Advanced Energy Field Interventions

Advanced energy field interventions in Healing Touch Therapy involve sophisticated techniques to manipulate and balance the body's energy field. These interventions are designed to address deep-seated energy imbalances and promote profound healing.

One such technique is the use of energy vortices, which involves creating spinning motions with your hands to clear stagnant energy and restore flow. Another method is the use of color visualization, where you channel specific colors to different areas of the body to support healing. Each color has unique properties and can be used to address specific issues, such as blue for calming or green for balancing.

Other advanced interventions include working with the chakras, the energy centers of the body. Techniques such as chakra balancing, clearing, and activation can help to harmonize the entire energy system.

Additionally, incorporating sound healing with instruments like tuning forks or singing bowls can enhance the vibrational frequency of the energy field and support deep healing.

Consistent practice and continuous learning are essential to mastering these advanced techniques.

Seek out advanced training programs and workshops to expand your knowledge and refine your skills.

By integrating these advanced interventions into your practice, you can offer a more comprehensive and effective healing experience for your clients.

CHAPTER FIVE

HEALING TOUCH FOR SPECIFIC CONDITIONS

Pain Management

Healing Touch therapy is an effective complementary approach to managing pain. The therapy involves the use of gentle, non-invasive hand movements to manipulate the body's energy fields, promoting relaxation and reducing pain. Practitioners often use techniques such as "magnetic passes" and "hands in motion" to clear energy blockages and balance the body's energy flow. These techniques help alleviate physical discomfort by enhancing the body's natural healing processes.

For chronic pain sufferers, Healing Touch can provide significant relief by addressing underlying energy imbalances. Patients often report a reduction in pain levels and an improvement in their overall sense of well-being after sessions. The therapy can be particularly beneficial for conditions such as arthritis, fibromyalgia, and migraines, where traditional pain management methods may have limited effectiveness. Regular Healing Touch sessions can help maintain pain relief, reduce dependency on medication, and improve quality of life.

Stress And Anxiety Relief

Stress and anxiety are common issues that can significantly impact one's health and quality of life. Healing Touch therapy offers a holistic approach to alleviating these conditions by promoting relaxation and restoring balance to the body's energy system.

During a session, practitioners use specific techniques to calm the mind and soothe the nervous system. This may include light touch or hovering the hands above the body to clear energy congestion and create a sense of tranquility.

Patients experiencing stress and anxiety often feel immediate relief during a Healing Touch session. The therapy helps to lower cortisol levels, the hormone associated with stress, and promotes the release of endorphins, the body's natural "feel-good" chemicals. Regular sessions can help individuals develop a greater sense of inner peace, resilience to stress, and a more positive outlook on life. For those with chronic anxiety, Healing Touch can be an invaluable part of a comprehensive treatment plan, complementing other therapies such as counseling or medication.

Enhancing Recovery From Illness

Recovery from illness can be a challenging and prolonged process. Healing Touch therapy can play a supportive role in enhancing the body's natural healing abilities and speeding up recovery. By balancing the body's energy fields, the therapy can improve circulation, boost the immune system, and enhance the body's ability to repair itself. Techniques such as "chakra connection" and "mind clearing" are often used to support the healing process.

Patients recovering from surgery, injury, or chronic illness often find that Healing Touch helps to reduce recovery time and improve overall outcomes.

The therapy can alleviate symptoms such as fatigue, pain, and inflammation, making the recovery process more comfortable.

Additionally, it can support emotional well-being, which is crucial for holistic healing. By reducing stress and promoting relaxation, Healing Touch helps patients maintain a positive mindset, which can significantly influence recovery.

Supporting Mental Health

Healing Touch therapy is not only beneficial for physical ailments but also for mental health. The gentle and nurturing approach of Healing Touch can help individuals dealing with depression, anxiety, and other mental health conditions. By working in the energy fields, practitioners aim to restore balance and harmony, which can alleviate emotional distress and promote mental clarity.

Patients with mental health issues often report feeling more grounded, centered, and calm after Healing Touch sessions. The therapy can help to release emotional blockages and traumas stored in the body's energy fields, facilitating emotional healing and personal growth. Regular sessions can enhance the effects of other mental health treatments, such as psychotherapy or medication, by providing a holistic and integrative approach to mental wellness. Healing Touch offers a safe and supportive space for individuals to explore and heal their emotional wounds.

Special Populations (Children, Elderly, Etc.)

Healing Touch therapy is adaptable to the needs of special populations, including children and the elderly. For children, the therapy can provide a gentle and non-invasive way to address issues such as anxiety, hyperactivity, and emotional trauma. Practitioners often use playful and engaging techniques to help children feel comfortable and relaxed during sessions. Healing Touch can also support children with chronic illnesses by alleviating pain and enhancing their overall sense of well-being.

For the elderly, Healing Touch can be particularly beneficial in managing age-related conditions such as arthritis, dementia, and mobility issues.

The gentle nature of the therapy makes it suitable for those with fragile health or limited mobility. Healing Touch can help improve circulation, reduce pain, and enhance the quality of sleep, contributing to a better quality of life for elderly individuals.

Additionally, the therapy provides a compassionate and nurturing touch, which can be profoundly comforting for those who may feel isolated or lonely.

In both children and the elderly, Healing Touch offers a holistic approach that addresses physical, emotional, and spiritual needs.

It supports the overall well-being of these special populations, helping them to feel more balanced, peaceful, and connected.

CHAPTER SIX

DEVELOPING YOUR SKILLS

Continuing Education Opportunities

Continuing education is essential for any healing touch therapist who wants to stay updated with the latest techniques and best practices.

Engaging in ongoing learning not only enhances your skills but also deepens your understanding of the body's energy systems. Numerous institutions offer accredited courses and certifications that provide comprehensive training in various aspects of healing touch therapy.

These programs often include advanced techniques, ethics in practice, and integrative approaches that combine healing touch with other modalities. By participating in these educational opportunities, you can ensure that your practice remains relevant and effective.

Workshops And Seminars

Attending workshops and seminars is another excellent way to develop your healing touch skills. These events offer hands-on experience and the chance to learn from seasoned practitioners and experts in the field. Workshops are typically focused on specific techniques or topics, such as energy balancing, chakra alignment, or working with specific populations like children or the elderly. Seminars, on the other hand, might cover broader themes such as holistic health or integrative medicine.

Both formats provide valuable networking opportunities, allowing you to connect with other practitioners, share experiences, and gain new insights that can enhance your practice.

Mentorship And Community Support

Mentorship is a powerful tool for growth in any profession, and healing touch therapy is no exception. Finding a mentor who has extensive experience and a deep understanding of the practice can provide you with guidance, feedback, and encouragement. A mentor can help you navigate challenges, refine your techniques, and develop your unique style as a practitioner.

In addition to one-on-one mentorship, joining a community of like-minded individuals can provide ongoing support and inspiration. Many professional organizations and local groups offer forums, meetings, and events where you can connect with peers, discuss cases, and share knowledge.

Building A Practice

Establishing a successful healing touch practice requires a blend of clinical skills and business acumen. Start by creating a welcoming and healing environment for your clients. This involves setting up a serene, comfortable space with soothing colors, soft lighting, and calming music. Consider the logistics of your practice, such as scheduling, record-keeping, and client confidentiality. Marketing your services effectively is also crucial; this might include creating a professional website, engaging in social media, and networking with other healthcare providers. Offering introductory sessions or workshops can attract new clients and build your reputation as a skilled practitioner.

Reflective Practices For Growth

Reflection is a key component of professional development in healing touch therapy. Regularly taking time to reflect on your experiences, both positive and challenging, can provide valuable insights and foster continuous improvement. Keeping a journal where you document your sessions, client feedback, and personal reflections can help you identify patterns and areas for growth. Engaging in reflective practices such as meditation, mindfulness, or supervision groups allows you to process your experiences and deepen your self-awareness. These practices not only enhance your skills but also contribute to your well-being, making you a more effective and compassionate healer.

CHAPTER SEVEN

COMMON CONCERNS IN HEALING TOUCH THERAPY

Addressing Skepticism

Healing Touch Therapy often faces skepticism, particularly from individuals accustomed to conventional medical treatments. This skepticism can stem from a lack of understanding or exposure to energy healing practices.

To address this, it is crucial to provide clear, evidence-based information about the therapy. Explain how Healing Touch works, its history, and its benefits. Share testimonials and case studies from clients who have experienced positive outcomes.

Additionally, offers educational materials, such as articles and videos, that highlight the scientific research supporting energy healing. By fostering an open and informative dialogue, you can help reduce skepticism and build trust in Healing Touch Therapy.

Managing Client Expectations

Setting realistic expectations is essential for a successful Healing Touch session. Clients may come with high hopes or misconceptions about the therapy. It's important to explain that Healing Touch is a complementary therapy, not a replacement for conventional medical treatment.

Discuss what clients can expect during a session, including the techniques used, the duration, and the potential sensations they might experience. Emphasize that healing is a process and may require multiple sessions to achieve the desired results. By managing expectations from the outset, you can help clients feel more comfortable and satisfied with their Healing Touch experience.

Handling Adverse Reactions

While Healing Touch Therapy is generally considered safe, some clients may experience adverse reactions. These can include dizziness, emotional release, or a temporary worsening of symptoms.

It is important to discuss potential reactions with clients before starting a session. Ensure they understand that these reactions are often part of the healing process and typically subside quickly.

During the session, monitor the client closely and provide support as needed. If a client experiences significant discomfort, adjust the session accordingly or pause the treatment. Following the session, encourage clients to rest, stay hydrated, and reach out if they have any concerns. By addressing adverse reactions promptly and compassionately, you can maintain a safe and supportive healing environment.

Ethical Dilemmas And Solutions

Practitioners of Healing Touch Therapy may encounter ethical dilemmas in their practice. These can include issues of client confidentiality, informed consent, and professional boundaries.

It is essential to adhere to a strict code of ethics to ensure the integrity of the practice and the well-being of clients.

Always obtain informed consent before starting any treatment, clearly explaining the process and potential outcomes. Maintain client confidentiality at all times, and ensure that any shared information is done with the client's permission.

Be mindful of professional boundaries, avoiding any actions that could be misinterpreted or cause discomfort to the client. If an ethical dilemma arises, seek guidance from professional organizations or experienced colleagues. By upholding high ethical standards, you can build a trustworthy and professional Healing Touch practice.

Legal Considerations And Insurance

Healing Touch Therapy practitioners must be aware of the legal considerations related to their practice. These can vary depending on the region and local regulations. It is important to research and understand the legal requirements for practicing energy healing in your area, including any necessary licenses or certifications. Additionally, consider obtaining professional liability insurance to protect yourself and your practice.

This insurance can cover legal fees and claims related to your services. Communicate the scope and nature of your practice to clients, ensuring they understand that Healing Touch is a complementary therapy.

By staying informed about legal considerations and securing appropriate insurance, you can operate your Healing Touch practice with confidence and professionalism.

CHAPTER EIGHT

FREQUENTLY ASKED QUESTIONS (FAQS)

What Is Healing Touch Therapy?

Healing Touch Therapy is a gentle, energy-based approach to healing that promotes balance and harmony in the body's energy system. Practitioners use their hands to gently manipulate the body's energy fields, intending to restore balance, reduce stress, and support overall well-being.

Unlike some other therapies, Healing Touch is non-invasive and can be performed with the client fully clothed. It incorporates a holistic approach, addressing physical, emotional, mental, and spiritual aspects of health.

The therapy involves a series of techniques where the practitioner's hands are either lightly touching or slightly above the body, following a specific sequence designed to clear, energize, and balance the energy system.

This can include techniques such as clearing energy blockages, balancing chakras, and supporting the body's natural healing processes. The aim is to facilitate the client's innate ability to heal and maintain wellness.

How Does It Differ From Other Therapies?

Healing Touch Therapy distinguishes itself from other therapeutic modalities through its focus on the body's energy system rather than physical manipulation or pharmacological intervention.

While traditional medicine often targets specific symptoms and diseases, Healing Touch takes a more comprehensive approach, seeking to address underlying imbalances in the body's energy.

Unlike massage therapy, which involves physical manipulation of muscles and tissues, Healing Touch is typically performed with minimal or no physical contact.

It also differs from acupuncture, which uses needles to stimulate specific points on the body; Healing Touch relies solely on the practitioner's hands and their intention to channel healing energy.

Another key difference is the emphasis on the practitioner-client relationship. Healing Touch sessions often involve a period of consultation and discussion, allowing the practitioner to tailor the session to the client's specific needs. This personalized approach helps ensure that the therapy is supportive and effective for each individual.

What Can I Expect During A Session?

A typical Healing Touch session begins with a brief conversation between the practitioner and the client to discuss the client's health concerns, goals, and any specific areas of discomfort or stress. This initial consultation helps the practitioner tailor the session to the client's unique needs.

Once the session begins, the client is usually asked to lie on a massage table, fully clothed. The practitioner will then proceed with a series of hand movements, either lightly touching or hovering above the body. These movements are designed to assess and balance the energy fields, clear blockages, and promote the flow of energy.

Clients often report a variety of sensations during a session, such as warmth, tingling, or a feeling of deep relaxation. Some may also experience emotional releases or a sense of heightened awareness. The session typically lasts about 60 minutes, although this can vary depending on the client's needs and the practitioner's approach.

After the session, the practitioner may discuss any findings or recommendations for further treatment or self-care practices. Clients are encouraged to drink plenty of water and take some time to rest and integrate the effects of the therapy.

Is Healing Touch Suitable For Everyone?

Healing Touch Therapy is considered safe and gentle, making it suitable for people of all ages and health conditions. It can be particularly beneficial for those experiencing stress, anxiety, chronic pain, or emotional trauma. Because it is non-invasive, it is often used as a complementary therapy alongside conventional medical treatments.

However, clients need to communicate any medical conditions or concerns with their practitioner before beginning treatment. This ensures that the therapy is appropriately tailored and that any necessary precautions are taken. While Healing Touch can be supportive of many health conditions, it is not a substitute for professional medical care and should be used as part of a comprehensive health plan.

How Do I Find A Qualified Practitioner?

Finding a qualified Healing Touch practitioner involves a few key steps. Start by seeking recommendations from trusted healthcare providers, friends, or family members who have experienced Healing Touch. Additionally, professional organizations such as Healing Touch Program and Healing Beyond Borders offer directories of certified practitioners.

When selecting a practitioner, consider their qualifications, experience, and approach to Healing Touch. It's important to choose someone who has undergone accredited training and certification, ensuring they adhere to professional standards and ethical guidelines.

Schedule an initial consultation to discuss your needs and goals, and to gauge your comfort level with the practitioner. This meeting can provide valuable insights into their communication style, professionalism, and ability to create a supportive healing environment.

Ultimately, trust your intuition and choose a practitioner who makes you feel safe, respected, and understood. A positive and trusting relationship between client and practitioner is crucial for the success of Healing Touch Therapy.